Nursing Assistant Journal/Notebook

nurse

{ners} n. a scrub wearing, smile bringing, life saving rockstar who lives to heal and loves to encourage.

See also: SUPERHERO

This book belongs to:

DATE: _____

DATE: _____

DATE: _____

DATE: _____

DATE: _____

DATE: _____

DATE: _____

DATE: _____

DATE: _____

DATE: _____

DATE: _____

DATE: _____

DATE: _____

DATE: _____

DATE: _____

DATE: _____

DATE: _____

DATE: _____

DATE: _____

DATE: _____

DATE: _____

DATE: _____

DATE: _____

DATE: _____

DATE: _____

DATE: _____

DATE: _____

DATE: _____

DATE: _____

DATE: _____

DATE: _____

DATE: _____

DATE: _____

DATE: _____

DATE: _____

DATE: _____

DATE: _____

DATE: _____

DATE: _____

DATE: _____

DATE: _____

DATE: _____

DATE: _____

DATE: _____

DATE: _____

DATE: _____

DATE: _____

DATE: _____

DATE: _____

DATE: _____

DATE: _____

DATE: _____

DATE: _____

DATE: _____

DATE: _____

DATE: _____

DATE: _____

DATE: _____

DATE: _____

DATE: _____

DATE: _____

DATE: _____

DATE: _____

DATE: _____

DATE: _____

DATE: _____

Quotes from Patients

Date

Who?

Where?

Quote

_____

_____

_____

_____

Quotes from Patients

Date

Who?

Where?

Quote

_____

_____

_____

_____

_____

Quotes from Patients

Date

Who?

Where?

Quote

_____

_____

_____

_____

Quotes from Patients

Date

Who?

Where?

Quote

_____

_____

_____

_____

Quotes from Patients

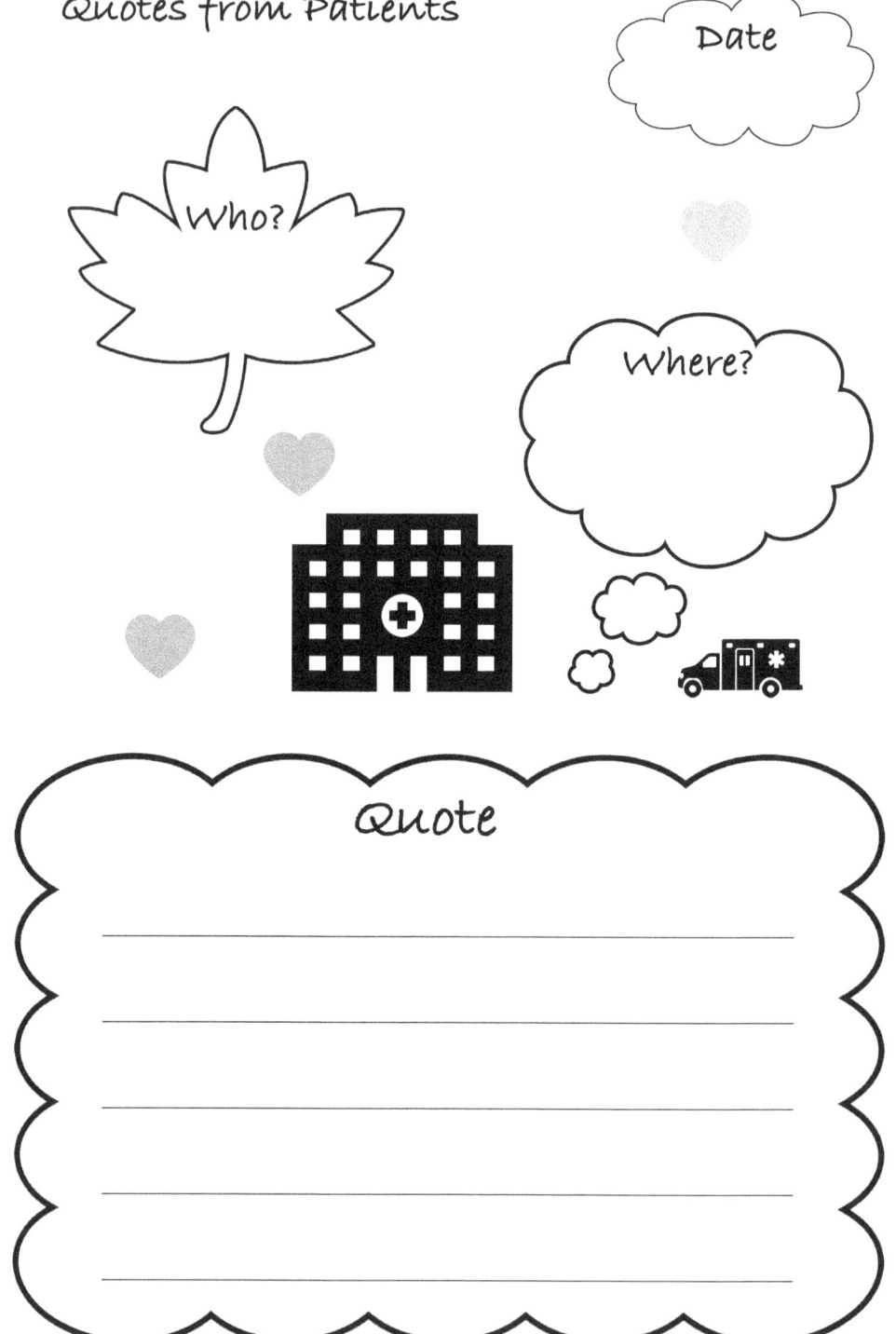

Date

Who?

Where?

Quote

_____

_____

_____

_____

_____

Coloring Section

I Had Fun Once, Then
I Went To Nursing School

Ativan A Nurse's Best Friend

Eat.
Sleep.
Nurse.
Repeat

DO NOT MAKE
ME SEDATE YOU.

Best Nurse Ever

I'VE SEEN MORE
PRIVATES
THAN THE ARMY
GENERAL

Nurse Squad

If You're Happy and You Know It, It's Your Meds

www.ingramcontent.com/pod-product-compliance
Lightning Source LLC
Chambersburg PA
CBHW070438180526
45158CB00019B/1623